explaining...
ASTHMA

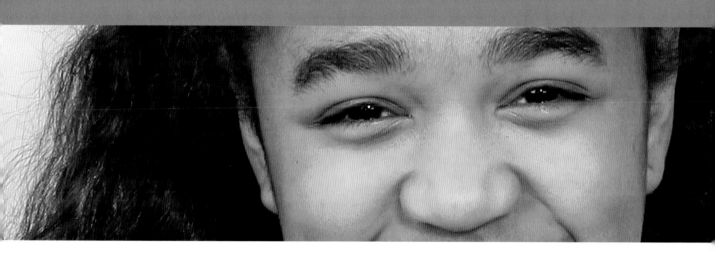

W
FRANKLIN WATTS
LONDON • SYDNEY

First published in 2008 by
Franklin Watts
338 Euston Road
London NW1 3BH

Franklin Watts Australia
Level 17/207 Kent Street
Sydney NSW 2000

© 2008 Franklin Watts

ISBN 978 0 7496 8261 3

Dewey classification number: 616.2'38

A CIP catalogue record for this publication is available from the British Library.

Planning and production by Discovery Books Limited
Managing Editor: Laura Durman
Editor: Annabel Savery
Designer: Keith Williams
Picture research: Rachel Tisdale
Consultant: Dr Clare Murray, Senior Lecturer and Consultant in Respiratory Paediatrics Royal Manchester Children's Hospital.

Printed in China

Franklin Watts is a division of Hachette Children's Books, an Hachette Livre Company.
www.hachettelivre.co.uk

Photo acknowledgements: Asthma UK: pp. 14, 18; Corbis: pp. 26 (Ray Morsch / Zefa), 31 (Ed Kashi); Discovery Picture Library: front cover top & bottom left (Chris Fairclough), pp. 20, 23, 24 (Chris Fairclough), 25 (Chris Fairclough), 30 (Bobby Humphrey); Getty Images: p. 12 (Christopher Furlong); Istockphoto: pp.13, 19, 21 (Anna Chelnokova), 28 & front cover bottom right (Peter Elvidge), 32 (Chris Rogers), 33 (Lisa Eastman), 34, 35 (Wendy Shiao), 36 (Branislav Ostojic); John Birdsall/www.johnbirdsall.co.uk: pp. 8, 39; Library of Congress: p. 10; Rich Clarkson: p. 37; Science and Society Picture Library: p. 11 (Science Museum); Science Photo Library: pp. 9 (BSIP, Laurent, Garnier), 22 (Andrew Syned); Shutterstock: p. 27 (Nigel Carse)

Source credits: We would like to thank the following for their contribution:
Jim and Ann Ryun (www.jimryun.com/www.ryunrunning.com)

Please note the case studies in this book are either true life stories or based on true life stories.

The pictures in the book feature a mixture of adults and children with and without asthma. Some of the photographs feature models, and it should not be implied that they have asthma.

Contents

8 What is asthma?

10 History of asthma

12 Increase in asthma

14 Who has asthma?

16 Healthy lungs

18 How asthma affects the lungs

20 What triggers asthma?

22 Asthma and allergies

24 Diagnosing asthma

26 Preventing an attack

28 Relieving an attack

30 What to do during an attack

32 Growing up with asthma

34 Living with asthma

36 Asthma and exercise

38 Future for asthma

40 Glossary

42 Further information

44 Index

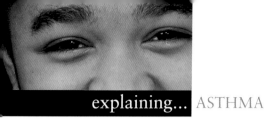

What is asthma?

Asthma is a condition that affects people's breathing because it narrows the tubes in the lungs, making it difficult for someone to breathe in and out.

Symptoms

There are lots of symptoms of asthma, although many people with asthma do not experience all of them. Coughing is one of the most common symptoms and most people with asthma sometimes make a wheezing sound in their chest as they breathe. Some people with asthma become short of breath more quickly than others when they exercise, and they may also experience a tight feeling in their chest.

▼ *You cannot tell whether any of these young people have asthma just by looking at them.*

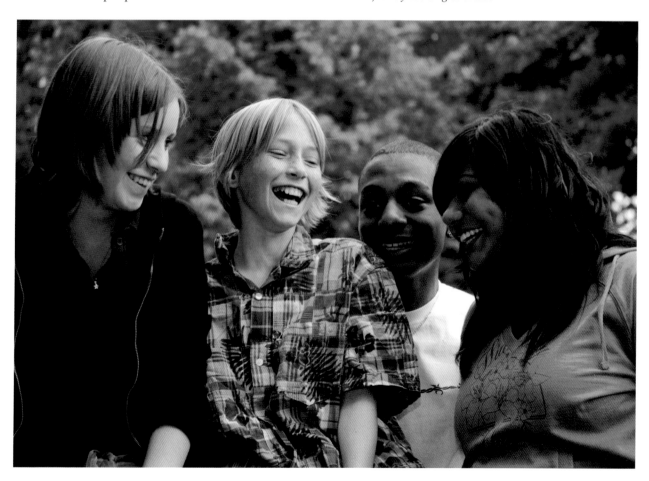

Asthma is not infectious so you cannot catch it from someone else and, if you have asthma, you cannot pass it on to your friends or other people you meet. People with asthma often cough to clear mucus from their airways and make it easier to breathe. This might sound as if they are ill, but they are not.

Same as other people

People with asthma look like everyone else and most of the time they can live like everyone else. They go to the same schools, play the same games and most can eat the same food. Asthma is a condition that can usually be managed by inhaling medication, so for much of the time, people with asthma can breathe with no difficulty. Sometimes, however, they may have an asthma attack. This is when their asthma becomes much worse.

An asthma attack

When someone has an asthma attack, they find it very hard to breathe in and out. They gasp for breath and can have great difficulty forcing air into and out of their lungs. Some people with asthma have more serious attacks than other people and may feel as though they are suffocating. In extreme cases, if someone has a very severe attack, it can kill them if they do not get the necessary medical treatment in time. People with asthma usually have special inhalers that they use to relieve the symptoms. An asthma attack can last anywhere from several minutes to several hours.

Asthma varies

Asthma is different for everyone. Some people have mild asthma and only have an attack occasionally.

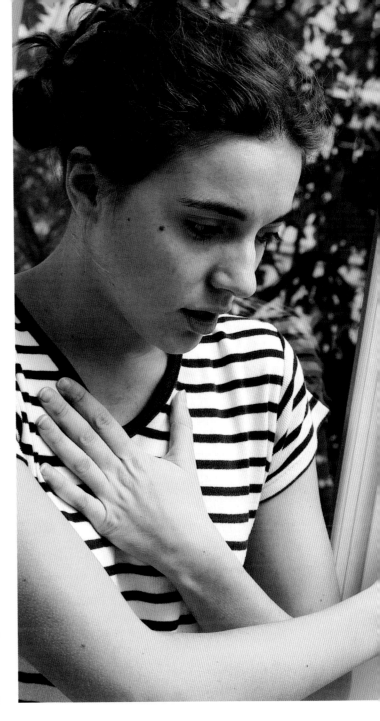

▲ *This girl is having an asthma attack. She is having great difficulty breathing in and out.*

Other people have severe asthma that affects many aspects of their lives (see Merriam's story on page 35). Some people's asthma is made worse by cigarette smoke, while other people are affected by household dust or pets. There are many different triggers that can cause an asthma attack (see pages 20–23).

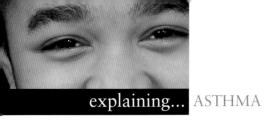

History of asthma

Asthma is not a modern disease. The first record of asthma appears in an Egyptian manuscript written more than 3,500 years ago, but it was Hippocrates, the Greek physician and philosopher, who first used the term 'asthma' about 2,400 years ago.

In Greek, asthma means 'gasping' or 'difficult breathing'. Similarly, the word for asthma in Chinese means 'wheezy breathing'. For centuries, doctors have struggled to understand and treat the condition.

HALL OF FAME

Many famous and influential people through history have suffered from asthma. They include:

Ludwig van Beethoven (1770–1827), composer

Benjamin Disraeli (1804–81), prime minister of Britain

Charles Dickens (1812–70), novelist

John F Kennedy (1917–63), president of USA

Che Guevara (1928–67), doctor and revolutionary

Martin Scorsese (1942–), film director

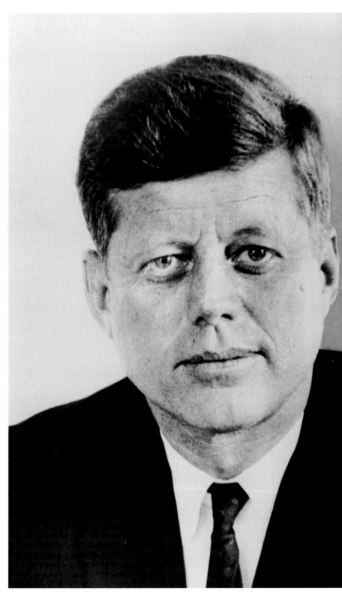

▶ *John F Kennedy was president of the United States from 1960 until his assassination in 1963.*

Early cures

From ancient times and throughout the Middle Ages, doctors thought that asthma was caused by an imbalance in the body. The Chinese used herbs, as well as acupuncture, exercise and diet, to try to restore the balance of the 'life force' within the body. The Romans recommended good diet, herbal remedies and prayer. In India, traditional doctors taught their asthma patients breathing techniques used in yoga and meditation.

Focus on the lungs

It was not until the late 17th century that two English doctors suggested that asthma was actually a condition of the lungs. Thomas Willis and Sir John Floyer both suffered from asthma themselves. Thomas Willis said that during an asthma attack 'the blood boils' and 'there is scarce anything more sharp or terrible than the fits thereof'. He suggested that the attacks were caused by a blockage in the bronchial tubes in the lungs, while Floyer said that they were brought on by a spasm of the smooth muscle of the bronchial tubes. At this time, however, no one understood what the function of the lungs was. They thought that breathing cooled the blood. Then, in the 1780s, the French scientist Antoine Laurent Lavoisier showed that breathing in oxygen, one of the gases found in air, was necessary for life.

Stethoscopes and spirometers

Two inventions helped doctors in their study of asthma. In 1815, René Laënnec invented the stethoscope, an instrument for listening to the heart and lungs. He got the idea after noticing children putting their ears close to the end of a long stick. They were tapping the stick and listening to the vibrations. By putting the hollow tube of a stethoscope onto a person's chest, he could hear what was happening in the lungs as they breathed. In the 1840s, John Hutchinson invented the spirometer. It measured the flow of air in to and out of the lungs. The spirometer used today is very similar to Hutchinson's original one.

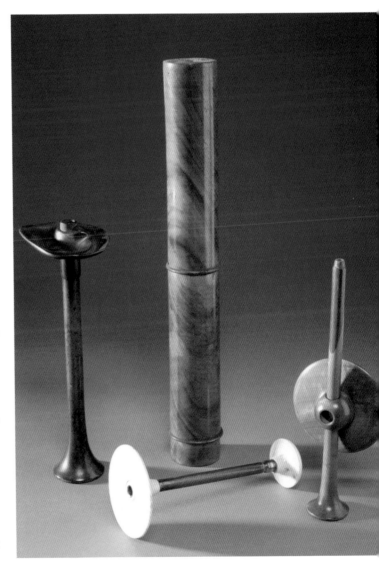

▲ *The large tube in the centre is one of René Laënnec's original stethoscopes. The others are later designs.*

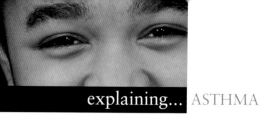

Increase in asthma

Asthma rates have increased rapidly in the last 50 years. In 1998, 17.3 million people in the USA suffered from asthma, but by 2004 the figure had increased to about 35 million, or about one in every eight people. In Britain, the number of people with asthma is now about five times higher than it was 25 years ago.

Around the world

The Global Initiative for Asthma (GINA) is an organisation that works with health-care professionals and public health officials to reduce asthma around the world. It estimates that today 300 million people worldwide have asthma.

Different countries

Asthma is much more common in developed countries than in developing countries. In undeveloped areas like rural Africa, asthma is quite unusual. In contrast, Australia has one of the highest rates of asthma, with just over one in six children suffering from it. Asthma in developed countries is probably now diagnosed more accurately than it was before, but this does not explain such a large increase.

It seems that the way of life in developed countries is making asthma more common, but people do not know exactly why this is. One example of this is given by GINA who have found that the rate of

asthma doubles when people migrate from the undeveloped Pacific Islands to developed countries like New Zealand. Asthma attacks are usually triggered by something in the environment (see pages 20-23), and so many studies have concentrated on how the environment in developed countries has changed in the last 30 to 40 years.

Air pollution

Some researchers are looking into the possibility that air pollution could be one cause of the rise in asthma. Most air pollution in developed countries

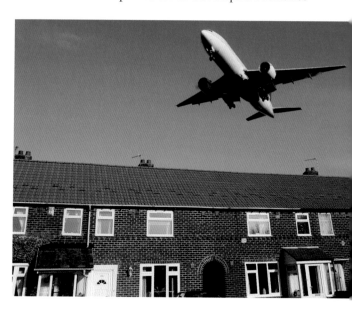

▶ *A plane coming in to land. People who live near airports are 57 per cent more likely to suffer from asthma. This may be triggered by air pollution from aircraft fuel.*

DIVIDED GERMANY

Between 1949 and 1990 Germany was split into two countries, East Germany and West Germany. Most West Germans lived in cities, while East Germany was largely rural. At that time, asthma was much less common in East Germany than in West Germany. In 1990 the two countries united. East Germany quickly changed and its people adopted West Germany's way of life. By 2004, asthma was almost as common in the former East Germany as in West Germany. This change in lifestyle probably caused the rise in asthma.

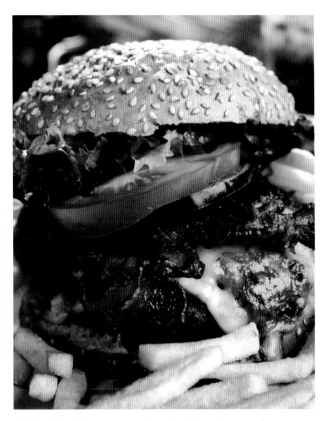

▲ *People today eat more fast food than they used to. This might be a cause of the increase in asthma rates.*

comes from traffic fumes, which contain gases that irritate the lungs and make it more difficult to breathe. In some large cities in developing countries, like Mexico City, both traffic levels and asthma rates have increased. However, it is still not certain that air pollution causes asthma, because, even in places where air pollution has decreased, asthma has still increased.

Air inside homes is polluted too, by dust, moulds and chemicals in products such as household cleaners and air fresheners. Today, children spend more time indoors, watching television and playing on computers, than children did 25 years ago, and so they are more exposed to these pollutants.

Other possible causes

Today, many people in developed countries eat much more fast and ready-made food than they did in the past. It is possible that this change in diet, possibly resulting in a lower intake of vitamins and minerals, has led to an increase in asthma.

Another possibility is that children are now too healthy and their homes are too clean! Although it is good to be clean, it means that children are not exposed to so many germs. The body's defence system works all the time, keeping germs out of our bodies and attacking them when they do get in so that they do not make us ill. If the body has fewer germs to fight it may begin to react to ordinary things as if they were germs, making allergies (see page 15) and asthma more likely.

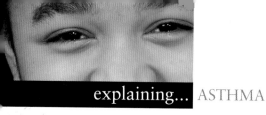

Who has asthma?

It is difficult to predict exactly who will have asthma, but some people are more likely to suffer from asthma than others. Most people develop the condition when they are young, others develop it much later in life.

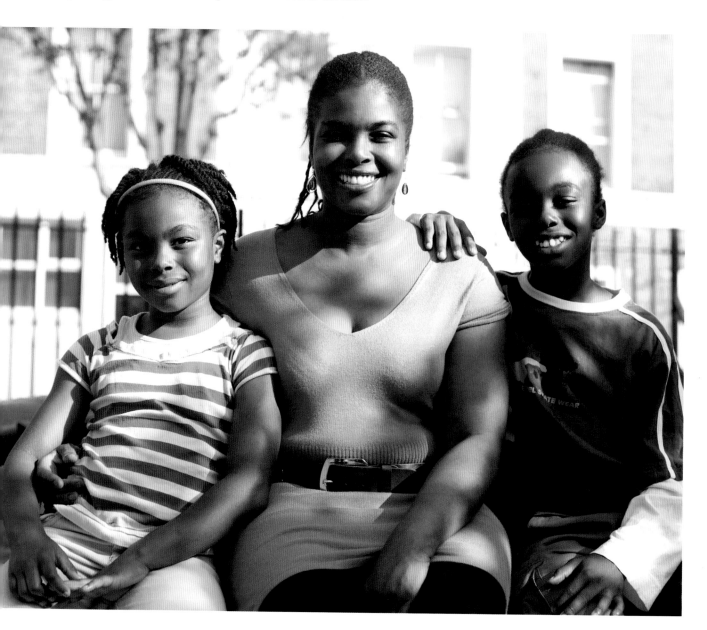

Families

Asthma tends to run in families. Everything you inherit from your parents is carried in your genes – half of your genes come from your mother and half from your father. Genes determine the colour of your hair and eyes and many other things about the way you look. They control how each cell in the body works and how your whole body grows and develops. There are several genes involved in asthma, which makes it harder for scientists to understand and predict how it may be passed from parents to children. If one or both parents have asthma or any allergies, their children are likely to develop them too. However, people whose parents do not have asthma or allergies can also develop asthma.

Allergies

Asthma and some allergies are closely related. You are allergic to something when your body reacts to it as though it were harmful, despite the fact that it is not harmful to most people. You can be allergic to things that you touch, eat or breathe in. If a person with asthma is allergic to something, it may make their asthma worse or trigger an asthma attack (see pages 22-23).

Smoking during pregnancy

When a pregnant woman smokes, the smoke she inhales affects her unborn baby. The children of mothers who smoke during their pregnancy are more likely to develop asthma. Research also shows that children whose parents smoke around them are more likely to suffer severe asthma.

◄ *Asthma often runs in families. In this family the mother and both of her children have severe asthma.*

JAY'S STORY

Jay is eleven and was diagnosed with asthma when he was five years old. Here his mum Kirsten talks about his condition and remembers the day that Jay had his worst ever asthma attack.

'I suppose it was always on the cards that Jay might have asthma. His dad is also allergic to pollen and to dust.

Jay's worst asthma attack was last spring. It was a cool, sunny day and he was playing in the yard with a friend. His friend called me outside because he was gasping for breath. His shoulders were up, and he looked like he was trying to open his lungs up. I tried not to panic, like I have in the past, and remembered what the doctor had told us. I calmed him down and gave him his inhaler.'

Kirsten says that trying to explain why is the hardest part of having a child with asthma. 'Jay can't understand why he has asthma when his friends don't. He asks us "Will I always have it?" We can't avoid the things he's allergic to – they are all around him at home and school. On the days when his asthma is bad he gets upset and irritable and doesn't enjoy school.'

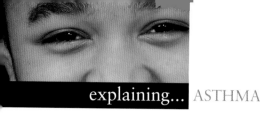

Healthy lungs

When you breathe in through your nose or mouth, the air goes into your windpipe, or trachea. From here, it goes through the bronchial tubes that branch out into smaller and smaller tubes inside each lung.

Airways

Each breath of air passes from the trachea into the bronchial tubes and so into the two lungs, one on each side of your chest. At the very end of the bronchial tubes are tiny balloons, called alveoli.

When you breathe in, the alveoli stretch and fill with air, and oxygen passes through the walls of the alveoli into tiny blood vessels. Your body needs oxygen to get energy from food. As your body burns the energy in food, it makes a waste gas called carbon dioxide. This passes from the blood into the air in the alveoli and is pushed out of your body when you breathe out. The alveoli are arranged in groups, called lobules.

Breathing muscles

You breathe automatically, using muscles between your ribs and a large muscle below your lungs called the diaphragm. When you breathe in, the muscles between your ribs pull your ribs upwards. At the same time, the diaphragm muscle pushes downwards. This creates space inside your lungs, which fills with air. When you breathe out, the opposite happens. The muscles between your ribs relax and the diaphragm rises, pushing air out of your lungs.

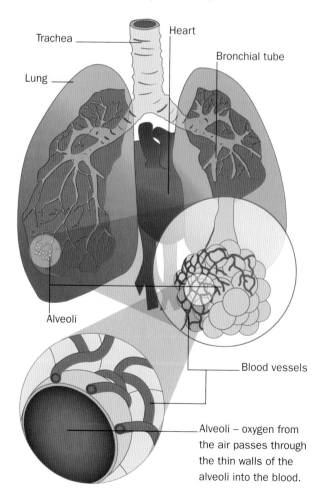

Trachea

Heart

Bronchial tube

Lung

Alveoli

Blood vessels

Alveoli – oxygen from the air passes through the thin walls of the alveoli into the blood.

◀ *The air you breathe in passes through smaller and smaller tubes to the alveoli, where oxygen from the air passes into your blood and carbon dioxide from your blood passes into your lungs.*

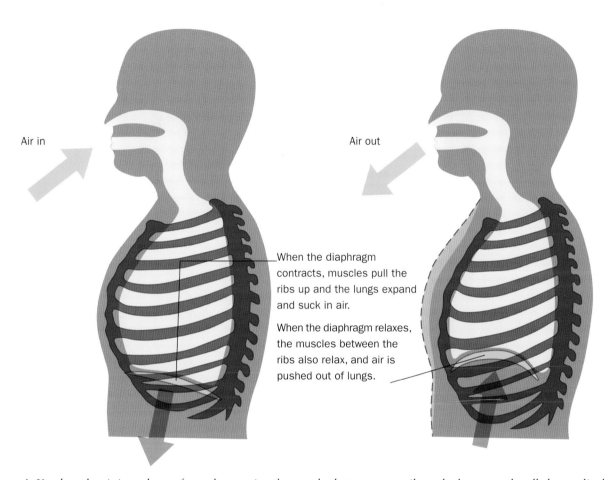

Air in

Air out

When the diaphragm contracts, muscles pull the ribs up and the lungs expand and suck in air.

When the diaphragm relaxes, the muscles between the ribs also relax, and air is pushed out of lungs.

▲ *You breathe air in and out of your lungs using the muscles between your ribs and a large muscle called your diaphragm.*

Healthy lungs

When you breathe in air, you also breathe in dust, germs and other things that pollute the air. The body makes sure these pollutants do not get into your bloodstream. The airways are lined with a thick liquid called mucus, which traps most of the pollutants before they reach the alveoli. The airways also contain millions of tiny hairs, called cilia. They gradually sweep the mucus back up the tubes and out of the lungs. If any pollutants get through the airways, special cells in the alveoli attack them. Only if germs or pollutants get past these cells will they get into your blood.

COUGHING

Coughing helps to push mucus out of the bronchial tubes. When you cough, you force a breath of air through the airways and out of your lungs. As the air rushes out through your mouth, it may bring mucus into your mouth or throat. You may also cough if smoke or another pollutant irritates the tubes in your lungs.

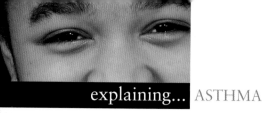

How asthma affects the lungs

When people have asthma, their airways, or bronchial tubes, are almost always red and swollen, making them narrower than normal. During an asthma attack, the airways become more inflamed and even narrower.

Sensitive airways

The airways of a person with asthma are very sensitive to particular triggers (see pages 20-21). If a person is sensitive to house dust and they breathe it in, their airways react to the house dust. The walls of the airways become more inflamed and they produce more mucus. The mucus is thick and sticky and so is difficult for the cilia to clear. Plugs of thick mucus can block some of the airways, making it hard to breathe.

Tightened muscles

The walls of the airways are surrounded by soft muscle. This is the same kind of muscle that surrounds your digestive tract and pushes your food through the digestive system. In your lungs, soft muscle helps the airways to stretch and contract as air moves in and out. During an asthma attack the soft muscle tightens up. This makes the tubes narrower and less able to let air through the lungs. At the same time, the lining of the nose produces mucus that blocks the nose, too.

▶ *The diagram at the top shows a normal airway, the one in the middle shows the airway of someone with asthma and the bottom one shows the airway during an asthma attack.*

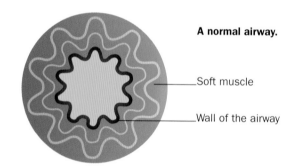

A normal airway.

Soft muscle

Wall of the airway

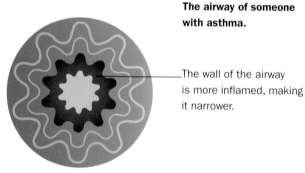

The airway of someone with asthma.

The wall of the airway is more inflamed, making it narrower.

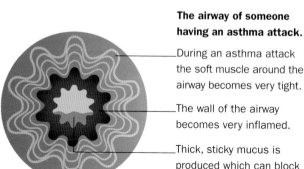

The airway of someone having an asthma attack.

During an asthma attack the soft muscle around the airway becomes very tight.

The wall of the airway becomes very inflamed.

Thick, sticky mucus is produced which can block the airway.

INFLAMMATION

Triggers cause an asthmatic's airways to become inflamed, making it difficult to breathe. Inflammation is part of the body's natural defence against germs, smoke, dust and other intruders. When part of the body is invaded, white blood cells and antibodies rush to the scene. They release histamine and other chemicals that make the affected part of the body swell and produce extra mucus. The inflammation and extra mucus help to protect the injured part while the white blood cells attack and dispose of the intruders. Insect bites and stings can produce a similar reaction in the body, causing a red swelling in the skin. Usually this is a good thing as it protects the body from infection, but, for asthmatics, inflammation of the airways is dangerous.

▼ *This is a photograph of magnified white blood cells.*
They have been dyed purple so you can see them.

AN ASTHMA ATTACK

Joshua did not develop asthma until he was nearly 30 years old. Here he describes what an asthma attack feels like:

'An asthma attack begins with a catch in the chest, a bit like snagging your clothes on briars as you walk along. My chest feels tight and breathing becomes more difficult – I have to work at my breathing, pulling the air in, pushing it out. If the attack gets bad, then breathing becomes really difficult and this can be worrying, because I am really struggling for air, but as much to get it out as to get it in. Then it's best to be still so that I need less air. At this stage my breathing sounds noisy, a hissing or even squeaky sound on the in-breath, and a moaning sound on the out-breath. Fortunately, my medication now stops the attack before it gets this bad.'

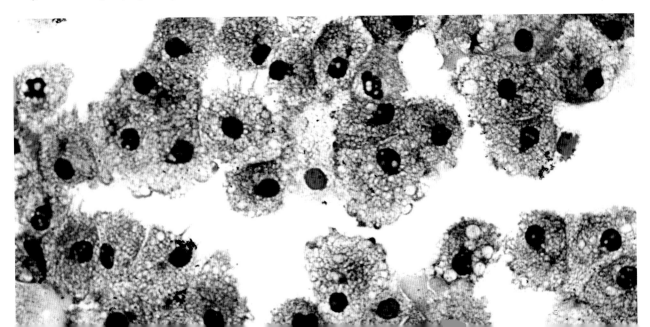

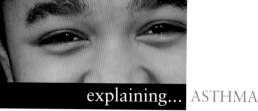

What triggers asthma?

Asthma is a condition that is always there, but most people do not notice it until they have an asthma attack. An asthma attack is usually triggered by something in the environment. There are two kinds of trigger – irritants and allergies (see pages 22-23).

Irritants are things that affect the sensitive airways in the lungs. They include cigarette smoke, cold air, chemical fumes and exercise. People who have asthma should keep a diary to note down when they have asthma attacks and what might have triggered them.

Cigarette smoke

When people smoke tobacco in cigarettes, pipes or cigars, they breathe out cigarette smoke. People nearby breathe in this second-hand smoke as well as smoke from the burning tobacco. This is called passive smoking and it is almost as dangerous to health as actually smoking the tobacco yourself. Tobacco smoke contains more than 400 chemicals, of which nicotine, tar and carbon monoxide do the most harm to the body.

Children are especially sensitive to tobacco smoke, because their airways are still growing, and children who suffer from asthma are the most sensitive of all. Tobacco smoking is now banned in all public buildings in many countries, making life cleaner and healthier, particularly for people who suffer from asthma.

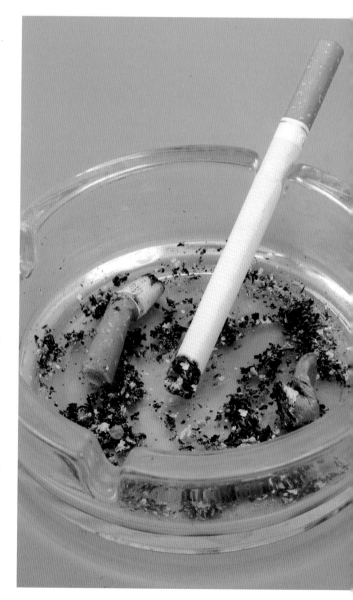

▶ *Smoke from a cigarette in an ashtray contains a higher concentration of poisonous chemicals than the smoke that is breathed out by a smoker.*

A DANGEROUS HABIT

Smoking affects the body in many different ways. The tar in tobacco irritates the lungs and causes coughs, particularly in people with asthma. The severity of the damage caused may take many years to appear. Smoking tobacco can cause cancer of the mouth, throat, stomach and, most commonly, of the lungs. Carbon monoxide from cigarettes clogs the arteries and causes heart attacks. It can also prevent oxygen reaching the brain, and can cause brain damage. Nicotine is a highly addictive chemical found in tobacco. It can cause blood vessels to tighten, making it hard for blood to travel around the body. Young people who start smoking may think that they can give up whenever they want to, but actually find it very difficult. Smoking can also damage the skin, causing deep wrinkles and making the skin an unhealthy colour.

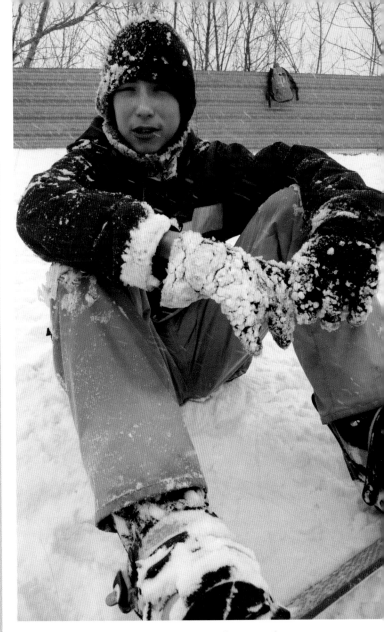

▲ *Breathing in cold air can trigger an asthma attack.*

Chemical fumes

Chemical fumes pollute the air inside and outside the home. Outside, traffic fumes and waste gases from power stations contain nitrogen dioxide and sulphur dioxide. In sunlight, some of the gases in traffic fumes combine to make ozone, a gas that can irritate the lungs and sting your eyes, nose and throat. Indoors, chemicals from household cleaners, air fresheners, hairsprays and other sprays can irritate the airways. More homes are draught proofed now, which also means that less fresh air comes in from outside.

Cold air and exercise

Cold air makes your airways contract. Most people catch their breath when they go out into cold air, but some people with asthma cough and wheeze too. Wearing a scarf over the mouth and nose helps to warm the air before you breathe it in.

People with asthma may quickly become breathless when they run about, and strenuous exercise can bring on an asthma attack. Exercise is good for everyone, however, including people with asthma, and so it is important for them to take part (see pages 36-37).

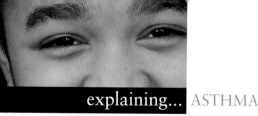

Asthma and allergies

A person has an allergy when their body reacts to something that is harmless to most people. Many different things cause allergies and they are called allergens. Allergens can make asthma worse, causing difficulty breathing, or cause an asthma attack.

What is an allergy?

Your body has several different ways of defending itself against germs and of getting rid of dust or other particles that you breathe in (see pages 17 and 19). However, when people are allergic to something, such as pollen, their bodies overreact. Most people do not notice if they breathe in pollen, but, if you are allergic to it, your nose will run, you may sneeze and your eyes may be sore and itchy. As the airways of people with asthma are already inflamed, further irritation will make their condition worse.

Allergens

The most common allergens to trigger an asthma attack are house-dust mites, animal dander and pollen, which are all breathed in. Certain foods and food additives, such as some preservatives and food colouring, can also trigger asthma attacks. Some asthmatics are allergic to certain medicines. In 2006, an Australian study showed that aspirin triggered asthma in about one in five adults with asthma.

▶ *This photograph of a house-dust mite has been magnified and coloured. Real house-dust mites are only about half the size of this full stop. House-dust mites can cause skin allergies and asthma.*

House-dust mites

You probably do not realise it, but you are sharing your home with millions of tiny house-dust mites. Much of the dust in your home consists of flakes of human skin, which you are constantly shedding. House-dust mites feed on these flakes of skin and they thrive in warm, damp places. Your bed could contain up to 1.5 million house-dust mites! They also live in carpets, curtains, soft toys and the soft coverings of chairs and sofas. It is not the mite itself that causes trouble, but its droppings.

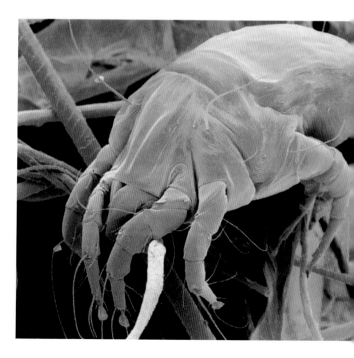

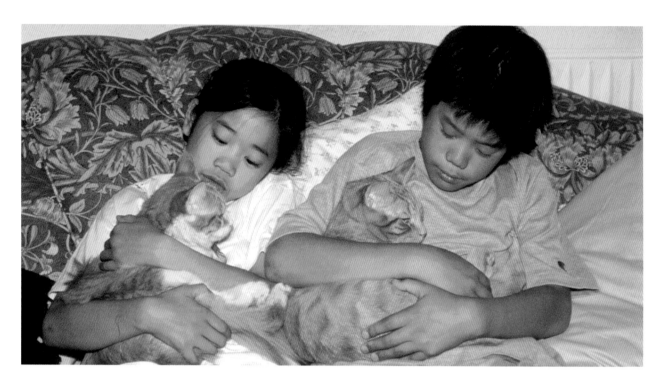

▲ *Many cats love to be stroked and hugged, but if you are allergic to animal dander you will probably have to keep away from them.*

Some people with asthma are allergic to them and they can trigger an attack. If you are allergic to house-dust mite droppings, there are several things you can do to avoid them building up in your home (see pages 34-35).

Pets

Many people are allergic to birds and furry animals, such as cats, dogs and rabbits. They can be allergic to their fur, feathers, saliva, dander and urine. Cats usually produce the strongest reaction, particularly in children, but rabbits, birds, dogs, horses and small mammals, such as guinea-pigs and hamsters, are also likely to produce a reaction in someone who is allergic.

Pollen

Pollen is the fine yellow dust produced by flowers. Inside each flower are unfertilised ovules. For an ovule to become a fertile seed, it needs to join with a grain of pollen from another flower. This means that pollen has to get from one flower to another. Colourful flowers rely on insects and birds to transfer the pollen from flower to flower, but plants with small, green flowers, such as grasses and many trees, rely on the wind to blow large amounts of pollen from flower to flower. Pollen is so light that it can drift for long distances. This means that in spring and early summer, the outside air contains lots of pollen. Hay fever is an allergic reaction to pollen. It causes itchy, swollen eyes and symptoms that are like a cold, including sneezing, having a runny nose and a headache. For some people with asthma, pollen can trigger an asthma attack.

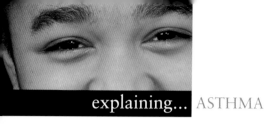

Diagnosing asthma

Asthma has to be diagnosed by a doctor at a local surgery or at an asthma clinic. Doctors diagnose asthma by asking the person about their symptoms and by measuring the flow of air into and out of the lungs.

Symptoms

Before a diagnosis can be made, a doctor has to find out which symptoms a person has, such as wheeziness, coughing, tight chest or breathlessness. They will ask whether the symptoms are worse at a particular time of day – or at night – and whether they are triggered by anything particular, such as stroking a cat or exercising. The doctor will also want to know whether anybody else in the family has asthma or allergies, or whether anyone in the family smokes. They are then likely to listen to the person's chest through a stethoscope to hear how well the

▼ *This doctor is asking the boy about his symptoms in order to diagnose whether he has asthma.*

person breathes in and out. It can take a while to diagnose asthma, particularly in very young children, as the symptoms of asthma evolve over time and may be mimicked by other things, like infections.

Peak flow

A peak flow meter measures how fast you can blow air out. You take a deep breath and then blow into the meter. You may have to do this three times to give an average reading. People with asthma cannot blow air out as fast as other people. How fast people can blow air out depends on their age, height and whether they are male or female.

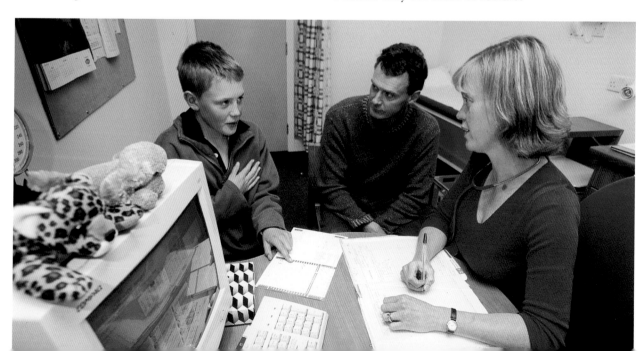

▲ *A peak flow meter measures how fast you can blow air out of your lungs. It is very easy to use.*

Once treatment of asthma has started, peak flow meters are a useful way of checking how well the medication is working. The person takes the peak flow meter home and is asked to take a reading at particular times of the day over several days. If the asthma is well controlled, the measurements should not vary much from day to day.

CASE NOTES

JASMINE'S STORY

Jasmine is 15 and was diagnosed with asthma when she was seven. This is what she says about being diagnosed.

'When I first had an asthma attack I was quite scared. I was outside at school and it suddenly got hard to breathe and my breaths sounded strange and wheezy. My chest felt really tight and like someone was squeezing it really hard. One of my friends told a teacher who made me sit down and breathe slowly. It took a while to stop because I was quite panicky. I went to the doctor with my mum the next day and she told him she thought I might have asthma. She said I had been quite wheezy at home. I had to breathe into a peak flow meter and he wrote down some things and talked to me a lot and asked lots of questions. He gave me two inhalers, a brown one to use when I get up and go to bed, and a blue one that I have to take around with me in case I have an asthma attack. He also gave me a peak flow meter to take home with me and I had to keep an asthma diary for a couple of months.'

Spirometer

A spirometer is only used in a doctor's clinic or surgery, and may not always be needed. The machine measures the largest volume of air you can breathe in and out and how quickly you can empty your lungs. If a person's asthma is brought on by strenuous exercise, a spirometer is used to measure the effect. Readings are taken before and after particular exercises, such as riding an exercise bicycle or running on a treadmill.

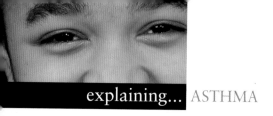

Preventing an attack

Doctors cannot cure asthma, but they can help people to manage the condition so that it affects them as little as possible. Two main kinds of medication are used. One prevents an attack and the other relieves an attack when it occurs. Both types of medication are taken by breathing them directly into the lungs, using an inhaler. Each kind of inhaler is a different colour.

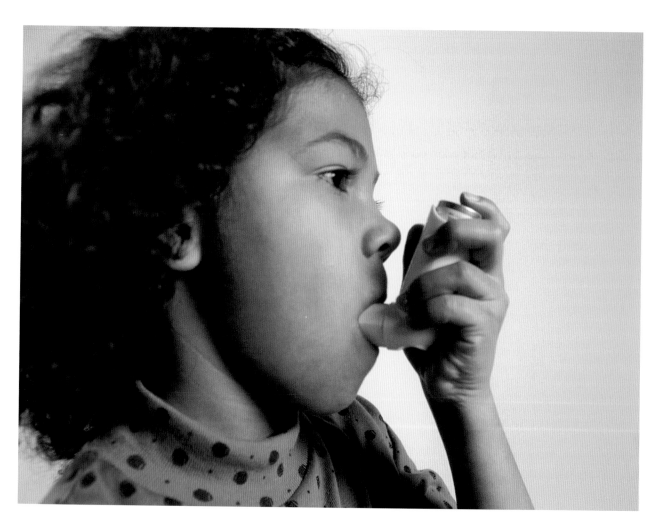

▲ *A young girl using a preventer inhaler. The drugs go straight into her lungs.*

Preventer inhaler

Preventer inhalers are usually brown, beige, orange or red. They contain drugs that reduce inflammation in the airways in the lungs. They reduce the swelling in the walls of the airways so that the bronchial tubes do not become so narrow, and they stop the airway walls producing so much mucus. This means that the airways are less likely to become blocked. If the person breathes in something that normally irritates the airways, such as traffic fumes, smoke or chemicals, the drugs make it less likely that this will lead to an asthma attack.

USING AN INHALER

There are several designs of inhaler. In the design shown here, the inhaler comes with the drug already in it. The person shakes the inhaler, breathes out and puts the mouthpiece in their mouth. They push the top of the inhaler down to release a dose of the drug and, at the same time, breathe in slowly and deeply. The person then holds their breath to give the drug time to reach all the airways.

ALEX'S STORY

Alex is 13 and has had asthma since he was six and a half. He uses a reliever inhaler and a preventer inhaler. This is what he says about managing asthma:

'I don't really think about it much because I follow the routine of using the inhalers which we've found works for me. You could say I treat asthma as a challenge, not a hindrance. It's just part of me. I have got into a routine for taking my inhalers and having check-ups. It is chest infections, coughs and colds that mostly trigger my asthma, so I try to avoid them! I also try to eat well and do plenty of exercise. When I get ill, I use my preventer two or three times a day. I only have to use my reliever inhaler occasionally, much less than when I was first diagnosed. It's difficult to remember what it was like before I was diagnosed and prescribed the inhalers, but having an inhaler and knowing how to manage your asthma gives you more peace of mind. You have to be aware of your asthma, but you should try not to dwell on it. Control your asthma, don't let it control you!'

Night and morning

People who have asthma are usually told to use their preventer inhaler even though they may have no symptoms of asthma at the time. The drug does not act fast, but it lasts for several hours. It takes between five days and two weeks for the preventer drug to begin to work fully, which is why it should be used all the time, and not just when the person feels wheezy or has a tight chest.

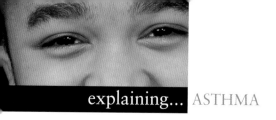
Relieving an attack

Although using a preventer inhaler will help to stop asthma attacks occurring, an attack can still be triggered. Then muscles in the walls of the airways tighten and the person has to use a reliever inhaler to make the muscles relax.

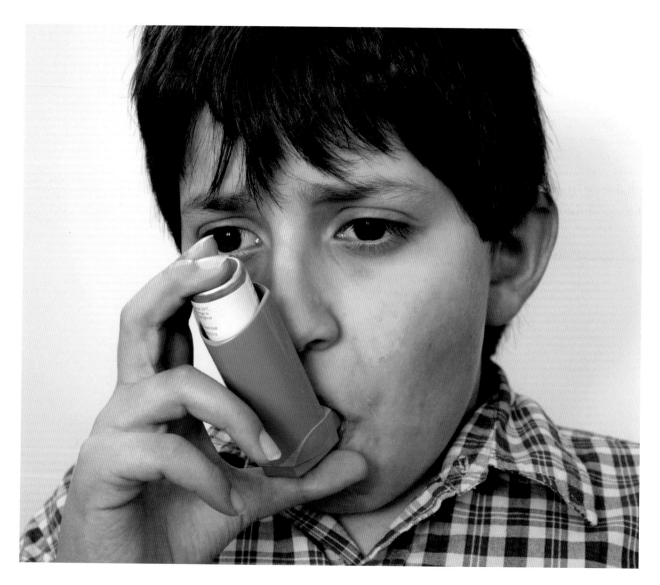

▲ *This boy is using an MDI inhaler (see page 29) to relieve an asthma attack.*

Reliever inhalers

A reliever inhaler is usually blue or grey and it contains a type of drug called a bronchiodilator. It relaxes the muscles in the walls of the airways, making it easier to breathe. Bronchiodilators act quickly, taking only a few minutes to start relieving an attack. The medication usually lasts for about four to five hours, although some relievers last for up to 12 hours. The advantage of an inhaler is that the drug goes straight into the lungs and does not affect the rest of the body. When you swallow a tablet or drink medicine on the other hand, it has to be digested and carried through your body in your blood.

Types of inhaler

There are several types of inhalers. A metered dose inhaler (MDI) releases a dose of the medicine when the top of the inhaler is pushed down. The person using it has to be able to co-ordinate pushing down the top with breathing in deeply. Some people find this difficult and may prefer to use a breath-activated MDI. This inhaler is a bit larger than the standard MDI. It still delivers a metered dose of medicine, but only does so when the person breathes in through the mouthpiece. Young children, who find MDIs hard to use, often use a spacer as well (see page 32).

A dry powder inhaler delivers the drug as a powder, instead of as a gas. The person has to breathe in hard to get the powder into their lungs and so they are not usually very suitable for young children. Dry powder inhalers are made in various shapes and sizes.

ADRENALINE

Bronchiodilators act like adrenaline. This is a hormone that is produced naturally by the adrenal glands. It acts to keep the muscles of your airways relaxed and your airways open. It also affects how fast your heart beats. Adrenaline works very fast in an emergency. If you are suddenly alarmed, your body releases extra adrenaline. It relaxes your airways even further so that you breathe more deeply. It also makes your heart beat faster and sends blood to your muscles so that you are instantly ready to deal with the emergency. Bronchiodilators are more specific than adrenaline. They work in a specific area and do not travel all over the body. This means they are safe to use many times a day and do not have side effects.

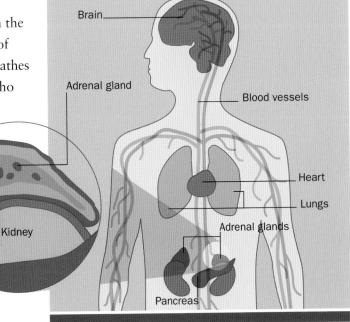

Brain

Adrenal gland

Blood vessels

Heart

Lungs

Adrenal glands

Kidney

Pancreas

What to do during an attack

An asthma attack can be alarming both for the person concerned and for those with them. If you have asthma, you need to know what to do if you have an attack. It is also helpful to know what to do if someone else is having an attack. The most important thing is for everyone to keep calm.

Using the reliever inhaler

People who have asthma should always carry their reliever inhaler with them. They should use it as soon as they feel an attack coming on. They should also sit down, and lean forward with their hands on their knees to support themselves – this is the most relaxed position for their chest. Then they should try to calm their breathing, by breathing more slowly and not too deeply. If the attack does not ease immediately, then the person should use the reliever inhaler again after a minute and continue to do this until their breathing begins

▼ *This boy is sitting in the best position to relieve his asthma attack. His mother is helping him to stay calm.*

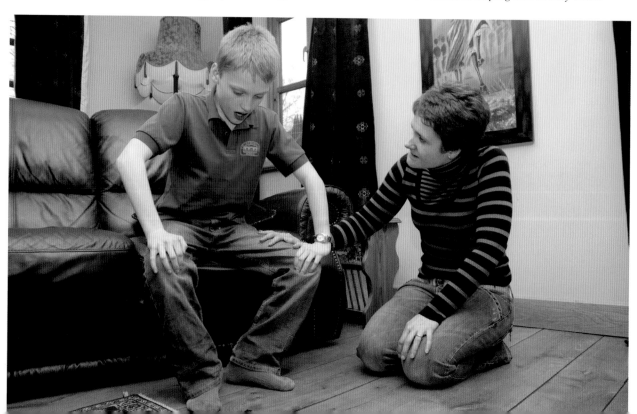

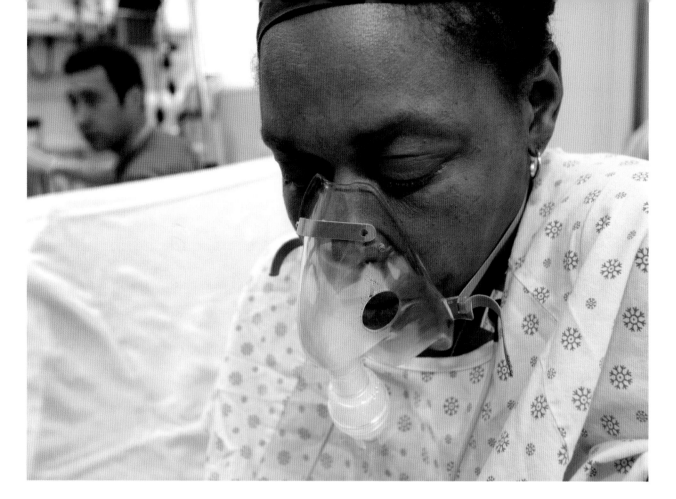

▲ *This woman is being treated for severe asthma in the emergency room of the San Francisco General Hospital.*

to improve. Coughing up mucus is one sign that the attack is beginning to lessen. The drug in the reliever inhaler should work in five to ten minutes, after which breathing should return to normal.

Helping someone else

When adults have an asthma attack, they should know what to do and so you just need to give them space and time to deal with it themselves. However, when young children, or people who are not prepared, have an asthma attack, you may need to calm them down and reassure them that everything will be all right. It is important to keep their chest open so that they can breathe more easily. This means that they should sit, rather than lie down, and you should not let anyone put their arm around them, because that constricts their chest. If they are wearing tight clothing, you can suggest that they loosen it. If the reliever inhaler has not worked after ten minutes, you should call a doctor or an ambulance.

Getting emergency medical help

If the reliever inhaler has had no effect after ten minutes, or if the person is upset, exhausted or cannot speak, they should be seen by a doctor or be taken to hospital. Here they may be given extra oxygen or their usual reliever drug that they breathe in through a nebuliser (see page 33). If the attack is very severe, they will probably be given stronger drugs, usually through a drip into a vein. In extreme cases they may even need to be put on a ventilator. This machine forces the right mixture of air into the lungs until the person can breathe on their own again. They will have to stay in hospital until their breathing has returned to normal.

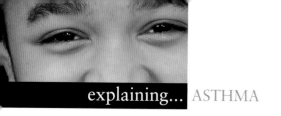

Growing up with asthma

Most people with asthma develop the condition when they are children. About half of all people with asthma have symptoms by the time they are ten years old and many children are younger than six years old when they have their first attack.

Asthma is not uncommon among toddlers and even babies, although it is difficult to diagnose correctly in very young children. According to the Asthma Foundation of Australia, 'Children aged 0 to 4 years are the group that most commonly visits GPs or emergency departments or are hospitalised for asthma.'

▼ *A spacer makes it easier for young children to inhale asthma drugs. The reliever or preventer inhaler fits onto the end of the spacer.*

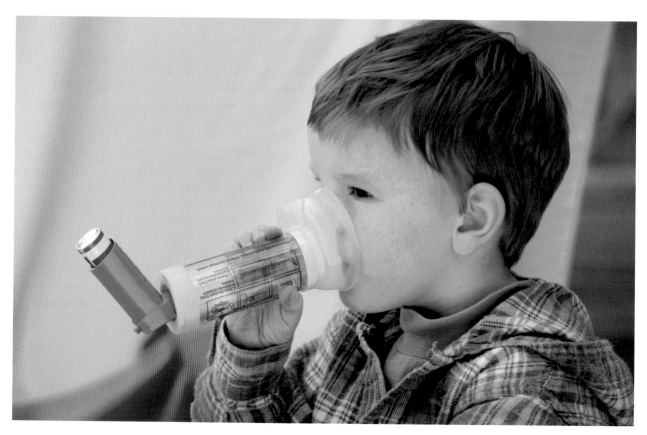

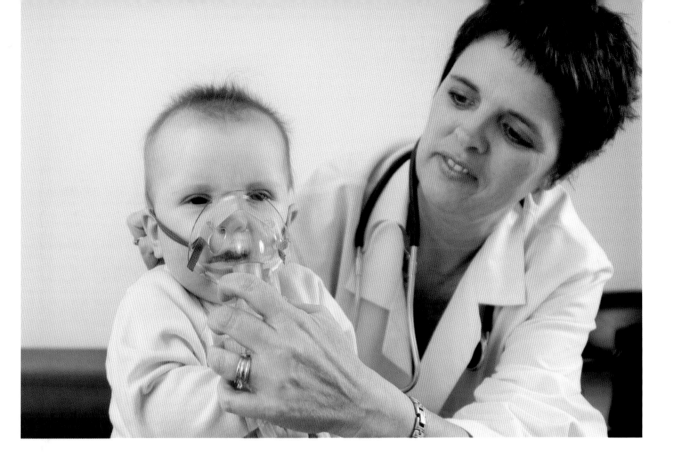

Treating asthma in young children

Asthma in babies and young children is treated with reliever and preventer drugs, just as it is with older children and adults. Young children, however, find it hard to use the same inhalers as older children and often use a spacer as well. A spacer is a clear plastic chamber that fits onto the mouthpiece of the inhaler. The other end of the spacer has a mouthpiece that the child can put into his or her mouth, or a mask that covers the baby's or child's mouth and nose. Instead of having to breathe in as the drug is released, the drug mixes with the air in the spacer. The child breathes in deeply and holds their breath. They then breathe out into the spacer before taking in another deep breath.

Nebulisers

If a baby or young child is having difficulty breathing, they should be taken to a hospital. They may be given medication using a nebuliser. This machine pumps oxygen or air through a liquid containing medicine. The nebuliser turns

▲ *This seven-month-old baby is breathing through a nebuliser.*

the medicine into a fine mist that is easy to breathe in. As with a spacer, children can breathe in the drug through the mouthpiece or through a mask. Using a nebuliser is the easiest way to get the medicine straight into the lungs, and so it is used not only with babies, but with people of all ages who are having a severe asthma attack.

Changing condition

Asthma changes from day to day. As a child gets older, it may become easier to identify the things that trigger an attack. The condition also changes as a child gets older and so it is important that parents and children work with their doctor to adjust the levels of medicine. Sometimes the condition has disappeared by the time the child is a teenager. This is more likely to happen with children whose asthma is mild. Even so, the asthma may return when the child becomes an adult.

Living with asthma

Most people with asthma manage their condition and live normal lives. They use their preventer inhalers as instructed by their doctors and carry their reliever inhaler wherever they go. They also try to avoid the things that trigger an attack. People with severe asthma have to be even more careful.

Avoiding triggers

Some triggers are easier to avoid than others. If you are allergic to certain foods or food additives, you need to check the ingredients before eating something. If you are allergic to certain animals, then you should try to keep away from them. Some triggers, such as traffic fumes and pollen, are much harder to avoid.

House-dust mites are one of the hardest triggers to avoid. If you are allergic to house-dust mites, you have to try to reduce the amount of soft furnishings in your home, as house-dust mites live in them. For example, it is better to have bare floors than carpets, and blinds rather than curtains. You need to vacuum frequently so that dust does not collect. You can get special covers for your mattress, duvet and pillow case that form a barrier between you and the house-dust mites in your bed.

At school

School teachers should know if any of the children in their class have asthma. In secondary school, the students are in charge of their own inhalers. In primary schools and nurseries, the teacher puts the reliever inhaler in a safe place so both the child

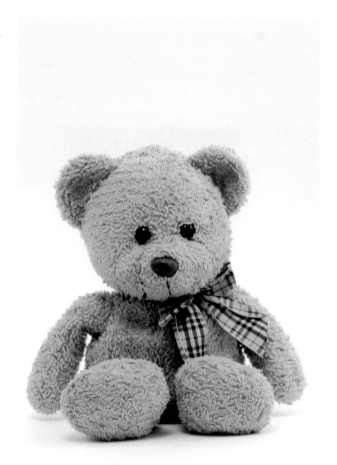

▲ *House-dust mites love cuddly toys. One way to get rid of them is to put cuddly toys in the freezer for at least six hours, because the cold temperature kills them.*

▲ *Children with asthma should make sure they have their reliever inhaler in their bag before they go to school.*

and teaching staff know where it is. Carol, a primary school teacher in London, says, 'The children know when an attack is coming on. It is usually when they are in the playground, so they tell a teaching assistant who comes with them to get their inhaler.'

MERRIAM'S STORY

Merriam lives in Johannesburg in South Africa. She has had severe asthma since she was born. She says:

'When I was a child I couldn't play normally like other kids. I had to take breaks – I had to sit down and breathe. I had to always carry a spray and sometimes I forgot it. My asthma is still bad. It is triggered mostly by rain – heavy rain brings down pollen from high in the sky – and by smoke. It is quite terrible at the moment because it rains more often in Johannesburg nowadays. I use a reliever inhaler and I take tablets prescribed by the hospital. I also have a nebuliser at home and at work. Asthma affects my social life. I don't like to travel far. For example, my friends went to Mpumalanga on the weekend. But I heard it was raining there. Also, because of the possibility of power cuts, I couldn't even take my nebuliser with me. So I didn't go. I can't go to social events, like parties, because of the smoking – smoke is terrible for me. I used to worry about my asthma. I thought that when I grew up it would go away. But when it didn't, I realised this is for life, so now I accept it.'

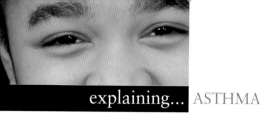

Asthma and exercise

Exercise is important, whether you have asthma or not. People with asthma should exercise regularly and can excel at their chosen sport. Although asthma attacks can be triggered by exercise, asthma should not prevent people taking part in sport, provided it is well managed.

Managing asthma

If you have asthma, you should always have your reliever inhaler with you when you exercise. Do warming up exercises before you start and, if you begin to get symptoms of asthma, stop exercising and use your reliever inhaler. Similarly when you have finished exercising, do some cooling down exercises, so that your breathing gradually returns to normal. If you know that exercise is likely to trigger your symptoms, then use your reliever inhaler before you begin.

▼ *People with asthma can play sport and compete in competitions if their asthma is well controlled.*

TOP ATHLETES

Many top sportspeople have asthma. These are just a few of them:

Paula Radcliffe, marathon runner

Tom Dolan, Olympic swimmer

Paul Scholes, international football player

Justine Henin, tennis champion

Dennis Rodman, basketball player

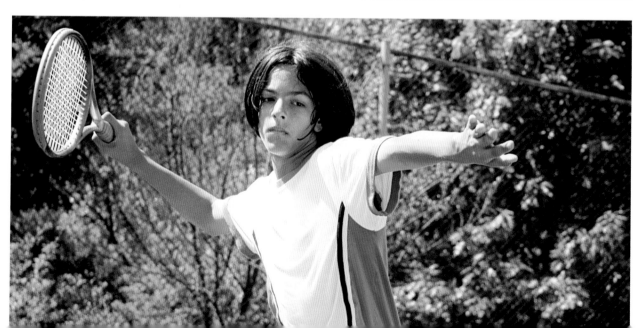

JIM RYUN'S STORY

Jim Ryun grew up in Wichita, Kansas and achieved national acclaim as a high school track and field star and as an Olympic medallist. He has broken three world records. He also has exercise-induced asthma.

'My love of running began when I tried out for my high school cross-country team. I not only made the team but went on to excel at the sport. I also realised I had asthma. Having not heard of exercise-induced asthma before, I thought my breathlessness during and after exercise was due to my lack of fitness. My coach recognised the signs and advised me to see an ear, nose and throat doctor, who diagnosed me with asthma. He also tested me for allergies, and it turned out that I had many that were contributing to my asthma. Once diagnosed, I was able to control my asthma and continue running.

I was the first high school boy to run the mile in under 4 minutes in 1964 and I held this record for eight years. I pursued my running career and went on to win a silver medal in the 1500-metre race at the 1968 Olympic Games. Now I organise running camps to train young athletes, some of whom also have exercise-induced asthma.'

You can learn more about the running camps that Jim Ryun organises at www.ryunrunning.com.

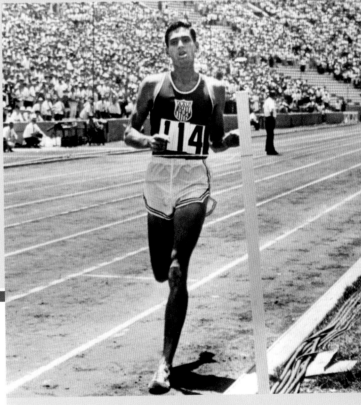

▲ *In 1967 Jim Ryun set the world record for the 1500 metres at the Los Angeles Coliseum, USA.*

Swimming

Swimming is one of the best forms of exercise for people with asthma, because the warm, damp atmosphere of a swimming pool is unlikely to trigger an attack. Swimming uses almost all your muscles and makes your heart and lungs work more efficiently. Swimming also encourages you to breathe deeply and evenly and so strengthens your lungs.

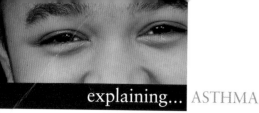
Future for asthma

Treatments for asthma have improved enormously in the last 40 years, but there are still many questions to be answered. Much research focuses on the causes of the condition and how it might be prevented. Today's asthma treatments manage and control the symptoms of asthma so that people can live a normal life. However, there is still no cure for asthma.

Unanswered questions

Scientists want to find out why asthma is increasing so rapidly in developed countries. Is there, for example, a link between diet and obesity and asthma? Is asthma caused by air pollution, and, if so, why should the Scottish island of Skye, which has very clean air, have the highest rate of asthma in the United Kingdom?

Researchers also want to find out when asthma begins. The children of women who used paracetamol while they were pregnant are more likely to be asthmatic, but does paracetamol cause asthma? The children of women who took large amounts of vitamin E during pregnancy are less likely to develop allergies. Is this significant?

Better drugs

The drugs available today work well for most people, but not for about ten per cent of people with asthma. For these people, the condition can be dangerous – about 180,000 people worldwide die from asthma each year. Research scientists are constantly trying to develop new and better drugs

for controlling asthma. Recent new drugs include LRTA (Leukotriene Receptor Antagonists), which reduces inflammation in the airways, and anti-IgE antibody therapy, which, although very expensive, can be used to treat allergic asthma.

More than anything, researchers are trying to develop a vaccine that will protect people from developing asthma, but this is still many years away.

DEVELOPING A NEW VACCINE OR DRUG

It can take up to 15 years and around £500 million for a pharmaceutical company to develop a vaccine or a new drug. By law, the company has to put new drugs or vaccines through several testing stages, from tests in the laboratory and tests on animals to several stages of tests on humans. The tests make sure that the vaccine or drug works and that it has no damaging side effects.

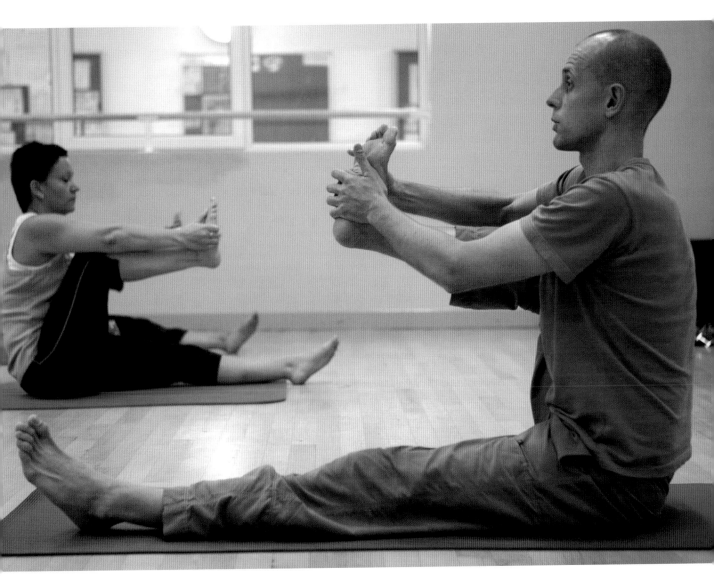

Complementary treatments

Some alternative medical techniques claim to lessen the effects of asthma in some people. One of these is a system of breathing developed by the Russian scientist Dr Buteyko. Many people with asthma, particularly severe asthma, have been helped using this method. Yoga is a system of movements linked with breathing that has been practised in India for many centuries. People with asthma have found that

▲ *In the past, Indian doctors used yoga to treat asthma. Today, many people find that some form of exercise helps them to manage their asthma.*

some of the exercises help to reduce their asthma attacks. However, Asthma UK says, 'There is little scientific evidence that complementary therapies are effective, especially used on their own.' They advise that you use them alongside conventional medicines.

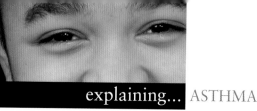

Glossary

acupuncture a technique developed in Chinese medicine that treats ailments and other problems by inserting special needles into specific places in the body

adrenaline a hormone that is produced in the adrenal glands; it opens the airways, makes the heart beat faster and prepares the muscles for action

adrenal glands parts of the body that produce the hormones adrenaline and noradrenaline

air pollution air-borne emissions, such as smoke and gases from factories, vehicles and power stations, that make the air dirty

allergy sensitivity or a reaction to something that is harmless to most people

alveoli tiny air sacs at the end of the airways in the lungs

antibodies substances produced by the body to fight infections and other intruders

bronchial tubes tubes that connect the trachea to alveoli in the lungs, also known as airways

bronchiodilator a drug that makes the muscles of the airways relax

cilia small, fine hairs that line the tubes inside the lungs

contract to become smaller or narrower

dander small flakes of skin in an animal's fur and feathers

diagnose to identify a disease or condition after careful examination of the body and symptoms

diaphragm a large sheet of muscle between the abdomen and lungs; when the diaphragm contracts, air is pulled into the lungs, when it relaxes, air is pushed out of the lungs

digestive tract a long tube which carries food through the body while it is digested and through which solid waste leaves the body

food additive something that is added to food, usually to improve its colour or taste, or to stop it decaying

hay fever an allergic reaction to pollen that can make your nose, throat and eyes itch and your nose run

histamine a substance that is released by the body when it is injured or invaded by germs or other external particles

infectious (of a disease) able to spread from one person to another

inflamed hot and swollen

inhaler device for breathing in medicine

inhaling breathing in

irritant something that causes irritation; it might cause redness, itching or swelling

meditation contemplation that stills the mind

metered dose inhaler (MDI) an inhaler that delivers a specific amount of drug

migrate to move from one place to live in another place

mucus thick, slimy liquid that moistens and protects organs' surfaces inside the body

nebuliser a device that changes medicine into a fine spray so that it is easier to breathe in

nicotine a chemical in tobacco that is highly addictive

ovule a female egg

oxygen an invisible gas in air that plants and animals need to survive

paracetamol a drug used to relieve pain

passive smoking breathing in someone else's tobacco smoke

peak flow meter an instrument for measuring the flow of air out of the lungs

pollen a fine yellow dust produced by flowers; pollen is the male sex cell

preservative a chemical that stops or slows down rotting in food or other organic substance

preventer inhaler an inhaler that contains medicine for preventing an asthma attack

reliever inhaler an inhaler that contains medicine for relieving an asthma attack

rural in the countryside

saliva a liquid made in the mouth

sensitive easily affected by something

smooth muscle muscle found inside certain parts of the body, for example, in the tubes of the lungs and the digestive tract

spacer a device that fits over the mouthpiece of an inhaler, making it easier to breathe in medication

spasm a sudden contraction of the muscles

spirometer an instrument that measures the flow of air into and out of the lungs

stethoscope a medical instrument for listening to the sounds of a patient's heart and lungs

symptoms changes in the body that indicate that a disease or other condition is present

trachea the tube that takes air from the throat to the lungs, also known as the windpipe

trigger something that sets something else off; for example, cigarette smoke can trigger an asthma attack

unfertilised (in plants) when a female ovule has not joined with a grain of pollen and so is unable to develop into new life

vaccine a substance given to improve immunity to a specific disease

ventilator a machine that takes over the function of breathing air into and out of the lungs

vitamin E a substance found in some foods, such as milk and oily fish, that the body needs to function properly

white blood cells cells in the blood that kill germs

yoga exercises and postures that promote control of the body and mind

Further information

Books

A Simple Guide to Asthma, Dr Eleanor Bull and Professor David Price, *CSF Medical Communications Ltd, 2005*

Asthma (Diseases and Disorders), Barbara Sheen, *Lucent Books, 2003*

Asthma (Health Issues), Sarah Lennard-Brown, *Hodder Children's Books, 2003*

Asthma (Just the Facts), Jenny Bryan, *Heinemann, 2004*

Asthma (Science: Health and Human Disease), Alissa Greenberg, *Franklin Watts, 2000*

Asthma: The Ultimate Teen Guide (It Happened to Me), Penny Hutchins Paquette, *Scarecrow Press, 2003*

Breathe Easy: A Teen's Guide to Asthma and Allergies (Science of Health), Jean Ford, Mary Ann McDonnell, Bridgemohan, *Mason Crest Publishers, 2005*

Breathe Easy: Young People's Guide to Asthma, Jonathan H Weiss, *American Psychological Association, 2003*

Coping with Childhood Asthma, Jill Eckersley, *Sheldon Press, 2003*

Living with Asthma (Teen's Guides), William E Berger, *Checkmark Books, 2008*

Need to Know Asthma, Jenny Bryan, *Heinemann Library, 2005*

Websites

www.aafa.org
Website of the Asthma and Allergy Foundation of America. Provides information about asthma, allergies, food allergies and more.

www.aanma.org/breatherville.htm
Part of the website of the Allergy & Asthma Network Mothers of Asthmatics, which tells you about how to cope with different aspects of asthma.

www.asthmaandchildren.com
UK website that helps to provide information and answer questions about children with asthma.

www.asthmaaustralia.org.au
Website of Asthma Foundation Australia containing information about asthma and links to organisations in different states.

www.asthma.org.uk
Website of Asthma UK, the main asthma support group for the United Kingdom. It includes general information about asthma.

www.asthmasociety.ie
Website of the Asthma Society of Ireland. It gives general information about asthma and personal stories of people with asthma.

www.ginasthma.com
Website of GINA, the Global Initiative for Asthma, with lots of information on World Asthma Day, and events planned in your country.

www.kidshealth.levinechildrenshospital.org/teen/
diseases_conditions/respiratory/asthma.html
This page on asthma from the KidsHealth website
contains lots of easy to understand information for
children about asthma.

www.lung.ca
Website of the Canadian Lung Association with
lots of information about asthma and their current
research projects.

www.lungusa.org
Website of the American Lung Association, part of
which gives information about asthma, personal
stories of people with lung conditions and links to
local organisations.

www.whatsasthma.org
Website containing a film that shows how the lungs
work, what happens during an asthma attack and
how asthma is treated.

Films

Asthma: Fighting to Breathe (Documentary)
Edge of a Dream Productions, 2003
A one hour documentary that gives viewers a closer
look at asthma.

Children and asthma (Documentary)
KQED, 2002
Part of a documentary series that look at the
reasons for the dramatic rise in childhood asthma
over the last 20 years.

The Motorcycle Diaries
FilmFour, 2004, Certificate 15
Film about Che Guevara's journey with a
friend through South America when he was a
medical student. Che suffered from asthma and
the film shows how asthma attacks affected
him and how they were dealt with in the days
before modern drugs.

*Note to parents and teachers: Every effort has been
made by the Publishers to ensure that these
websites are suitable for children, that they are of
the highest educational value, and that they contain
no inappropriate or offensive material. However,
because of the nature of the Internet, it is
impossible to guarantee that the contents of these
sites will not be altered. We strongly advise that
Internet access is supervised by a responsible adult.*

Index

adrenaline 29
Africa, incidence of asthma in 12
air pollution 12-13, 38
airways 8, 9, 11, 16, 17, 18, 19, 20, 21, 22, 27, 28, 29, 38
allergens 22
allergies 13, 15, 20, 22-23, 24, 37, 38
alveoli 16, 17
animals 9, 22, 23, 24, 34
asthma attacks 9, 11, 20, 30-31, 32
  effects 9, 11, 15, 18, 19, 25
  treatment 9, 19, 25, 26-27, 28-29, 30-31, 33, 35, 39
  triggers 9, 12, 15, 20, 21, 22-23, 33, 34, 36, 37
Australia 12, 22, 32

Beethoven, Ludwig van 10
breathing 10, 11, 21, 36
  allergies 15, 18, 22, 27
  breathing difficulties 8, 9, 10, 13, 18, 19, 21, 22, 25, 33, 35
  breathing techniques 11, 30, 31, 39
  exercise 21, 36, 37
  how we breathe 16, 17
  listening to 11
  measuring 24, 25
  medication 26, 27, 29, 30, 31, 33, 36
  oxygen 11, 16
bronchial tubes see airways
bronchiodilators 29

carbon dioxide 16
causes of asthma 11, 13, 38
children 11, 12, 13, 15, 20, 23, 24, 29, 32, 31, 33, 34, 35, 38
cigarette smoke 9, 20
cold air 20, 21
coughing 8, 9, 17, 21, 24, 27, 31

defence system 13
developed countries 12, 13, 38

developing countries 12, 13
diagnosing 12, 15, 24-25, 27, 32, 37
diaphragm 16, 17
Dickens, Charles 10
diet 9, 11, 13, 22, 34, 38
digestive system 18
Disraeli, Benjamin 10

environment 12, 20
exercise 8, 11, 20, 21, 25, 27, 36, 37, 39

family 15, 24
Floyer, Sir John 11
food 9, 13, 16, 18, 22, 34

genes 15
germs 13, 17, 19, 22
Global Initiative for Asthma (GINA) 12
Guevara, Che 10

hay fever 23
Hippocrates 10
house-dust mites 22-23, 34
household dust 9, 18
Hutchinson, John 11

infection 19, 24, 27
inflammation 19, 22, 27, 38
inhaler 9, 15, 25, 26, 27, 28, 29, 33, 34, 35
  preventer inhaler 26, 27, 28, 32, 34
  reliever inhaler 27, 28, 29, 30, 31, 32, 33, 34, 35, 36

Kennedy, John F 10

Laënnec, René 11
Lavoisier, Antoine Laurent 11
lungs 8, 9, 11, 13, 15, 16-17, 18-19, 20, 21, 24, 25, 26, 27, 29, 31, 33, 37

medication 9, 19, 22, 25, 26, 29, 33, 38, 39 see also inhaler and nebuliser
metered dose inhaler (MDI) 29
mucus 9, 17, 18, 19, 27, 31

nebuliser 31, 33, 35

oxygen 11, 16, 21, 31, 33

parents 15, 33
passive smoking 20
peak flow meter 24, 25
pets 9, 23
pollen 15, 22, 23, 34, 35
pregnancy 15, 38

research 12, 15, 18, 38
Ryun, Jim 37

school 9, 15, 25, 34-35, 37
Scorsese, Martin 10
smoking 15, 20, 21, 24, 35
spacer 29, 32, 33
spirometer 11, 25
stethoscope 11, 24
swimming 37
symptoms 8, 9, 23, 24, 27, 32, 36, 38

trachea see windpipe
traffic fumes 12-13, 21, 27, 34
treatment 9, 25, 38-39 see also inhaler, medication and nebuliser
triggers 9, 12, 15, 18, 19, 20-21, 22, 23, 24, 27, 28, 33, 35, 34, 36, 37

United States (USA) 10, 12, 37

vaccine 38

Willis, Thomas 11
windpipe 16

yoga 11, 39

These are the list of contents for each title in Explaining:

Asthma

What is asthma? • History of asthma • Increase in asthma • Who has asthma? • Healthy lungs • How asthma affects the lungs • What triggers asthma? • Asthma and allergies • Diagnosing asthma • Preventing an attack • Relieving an attack • What to do during an attack • Growing up with asthma • Living with asthma • Asthma and exercise • Future

Autism

What is autism? • Autism: a brief history • The rise of autism • The autistic spectrum • The signs of autism • Autism and inheritance • The triggers of autism • Autism and the body • Autism and mental health • Can autism be treated? • Living with autism • Autism and families • Autism and school • Asperger syndrome • Autism and adulthood • The future for autism

Blindness

What is blindness? • Causes and effects • Visual impairment • Colour blindness and night blindness • Eye tests • Treatments and cures • Coping with blindness • Optical aids • Guide dogs and canes • Home life • On the move • Blindness and families • Blindness at school • Blindness as an adult • Blindness, sport and leisure • The future for blindness

Cerebral Palsy

What is cerebral palsy? • The causes of cerebral palsy • Diagnosis • Types of cerebral palsy • Other effects of cerebral palsy • Managing cerebral palsy • Other support • Technological support • Communication • How it feels • Everyday life • Being at school • Cerebral palsy and the family • Into adulthood • Raising awareness • The future

Cystic Fibrosis

What is cystic fibrosis? • A brief history • What causes cystic fibrosis? • Screening and diagnosis • The effects of cystic fibrosis • How is cystic fibrosis managed? • Infections and illness • A special diet • Clearing the airways • Physical exercise • Cystic fibrosis and families • Cystic fibrosis at school • Living with cystic fibrosis • Living longer • New treatments • Gene therapy

Deafness

What is deafness? • Ears and sounds • Types of deafness • Causes of deafness • Signs of deafness • Diagnosis • Treating deafness • Lip reading • Sign language • Deafness and education • Schools for the deaf • Deafness and adulthood • Technology • Deafness and the family • Fighting discrimination • Latest research

Diabetes

What is diabetes? • Type 1 diabetes • Type 2 diabetes • Symptoms and diagnosis • Medication • Hypoglycaemia • Eyes, skin and feet • Other health issues • Healthy eating and drinking • Physical activity • Living with diabetes • Diabetes and families • Diabetes at school • Growing up with diabetes • The future for diabetics

Down's syndrome

What is Down's syndrome? • Changing attitudes • Who has Down's Syndrome? • What are chromosomes? • The extra chromosome • Individual differences • Health problems • Testing for Down's Syndrome • Diagnosing at birth • Babies • Toddlers • At school • Friendships and fun • Effects on the family • Living independently • Down's syndrome community

Epilepsy

What is epilepsy? • Causes and effects • Who has epilepsy? • Partial seizures • Generalised seizures • Triggers • Diagnosis • How you can help • Controlling epilepsy • Taking medicines • Living with epilepsy • Epilepsy and families • Epilepsy at school • Sport and leisure • Growing up with epilepsy • The future for epilepsy

Food allergy

What are food allergies? • Food allergies: a brief history • Food aversion, intolerance or allergy? • What is an allergic reaction? • Food allergies: common culprits • Anaphylaxis • Testing for food allergies • Avoiding allergic reactions • Treating allergic reactions • Food allergies on the rise • Food allergies and families • Food allergies and age • Living with food allergies • 21st century problems • The future for food allergies

Bret Hto
DGS ozlω

0 4 MAR 2015

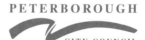